everything has become birds

everything has become birds

poems by

Peter Grandbois

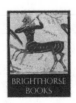

2021

Printed in the United States of America

Brighthorse Books
13202 North River Drive
Omaha, NE 68112

ISBN: 978-1-944467-26-5

Cover Art © Rob Clayton

Brighthorse Books is a small literary press based in Omaha, Nebraska, publishing books of poetry, short fiction, and novels.

For information about Brighthorse Books, visit us on the web at brighthorsebooks.com. For information about the Brighthorse Book Awards, go to https://brighthorsebooks.submittable.com/submit. Brighthorse books are distributed to the trade through Ingram Book Group and its distribution partners. For more information, go to https://ipage.ingramcontent.com/ipage/li001.jsp.

"We're all mad here."
THE CHESHIRE CAT

Contents

VI. THE MODERN ERA   73

everything has become birds

I
ANTIQUITY

"Those whom the gods destroy,
they first make mad."
EURIPIDES

Black angel

Madness begins as punishment. Saul punished after neglecting his
religious duty, Nebuchadnezzar for the sin of pride, Cassandra for
refusing to have sex with Apollo. The penalty—pollution of the mind.
The gods—or God—the polluter.

A crow in the snow

on the side of the road in

morning's haloed light

There is no shepherd but silence

"I shall soon make you dance more wildly and I shall play upon you a pipe of terror."
LYSSA, GREEK GOD OF MADNESS (FROM *HERACLES,* BY EURIPIDES)

Here in this light

each scattering
of stones

carries the sound
of a field

in winter

or a day
about to break

What can we do
but run

through
this dark labyrinth

between uprooted nights
that lie in wait

like prayer

Don't leave us here
in the space

between one stillness
and another

when all we want
is to be touched

again

Tell us we're yours
Make us live

on the edge
of this barbed wire
life

Promise we are
always almost

home

Against the broken stone

"But look, why am I anchored like a ship with ropes round my powerful chest and arms? Why am I sitting against the broken stone pillar with corpses all around me? Did I destroy my own house or was I possessed?"
HERACLES

Like a spider caught in a glue trap high on a shelf,
or a crow that flies into a narrow moon,

Like a liturgy of branches imploring the dark,
or an old law forbidding the sun,

Like the carnage of dandelion fluff
strewn about the grass,

We don't know how we got here.
This place was never promised.

Listen—there is always more to strip away,
more blood and broken bone to lose

before night folds in on itself and we wake
halved by the inarticulate darkness,

waiting for the signs to shower upon us,
possessed by a will wholly our own.

The biggest problems come from being

After night sinks into
its private stillness,

and you stand before a mirror
turned the wrong way,

remember that the world, too,
is exhausted, having devoured

everything it could from sky.
You'll need to look elsewhere

for something to hold you
together, lavender ice cream,

perhaps, or the neighbor's cat.
Considering how often

we must reinvent ourselves,
how many times we try to speak

the silent language of the Absent,
it's no wonder we choose to stumble

away from the one story worth telling.

The road out is like the road in

"Alas, poor men, their destiny. When all goes well a shadow will overthrow it. If it be unkind, one stroke of a wet sponge wipes all the picture out."
CASSANDRA

It's something like a bird
eyeing a petrified sky,

or a spider contemplating
the emptiness of shoes,

the way you wake each morning,
holding your breath,

before stepping into the undertow
of cold,

as if you could rephrase the question
dreamt in that other dark,

the need to understand why at sixteen
you and your friend took turns

holding on to the roof of the car
while the other spun donuts in the field,

each trying his best to lose.
You've got to choose something.

That sliding off into air, the choking dust
as you lie gasping on the ground,

seemed better than doubling back
to the wound buried deep within,

that other field we pray
will never be found.

Somewhere hidden

"My body is dead. I am the name it had."
ORESTES

Only I can't remember my name and
now I'm no more real than the hammering
from somewhere beyond the neighbor's
or the barks my dogs can't stop answering
this morning. I used to imagine
I could stand in a river of paper
and catch the secret of myself like a fish,
but there's inky darkness at the bottom,
and the barking goes on and on,
and no one is alive who gets buried
by the past, and our first dream is of
our name flying on the back of a dove
away from us and through the murmuring
rain, and who gives the dead a hammer.

II

THE MIDDLE AGES

"To know the face of God is to know madness."
LEOBEN CONOY,
BATTLESTAR GALACTICA

A candle lit in the hollow of a wall

The middle ages saw madness as blessed, a condition of increased spiritual insight. To see the unseen was divine. Reason alone could not approach mystery; therefore, the privileging of un-reason. "Faith is to believe what you do not see; the reward of this faith is to see what you believe." (St. Augustine, *Sermones*, 4:1:1)

Under sutured stars,

the sheerest slip of seeing

keeps us in pieces.

What certain voice

When I was a boy,
My mother sat me down
At the kitchen table
And said to me, "You are
The man of the house now."
My father had moved out.
My mother couldn't stop crying.

All I can remember thinking
Is that it would be like
Halloween. I'd already played
Dracula, Frankenstein, Wolfman.
What was one more part?
It's hard to see the exact length
Of childhood, or any other life
Shaped in this handmade world.

Forty years later, in a café,
The woman across from me,
The woman with whom I'd been
Having an affair for the past year,
The woman with whom I was planning
To leave my family asks, "Who are you?"
As if we could hold more than a guess,
as if whatever changing light
moves through us were a choice.

This is how you become absent

"But I saw these visions not in dreams, nor sleeping, nor in frenzy, nor with the eyes of my body, neither did I hear them with my exterior ears, nor in hidden places did I perceive them, but watching them, and looking carefully in an innocent mind, with the eyes and ears of the interior man, in open places, did I perceive them."
HILDEGARD OF BINGEN (1098–1179)

We cover our heads
And hold our breath,
Thinking that being
Alive is easy to imagine.

We live our lives
Waiting for the silence
Of evening sky
To fill us again.

We touch the ocean
Inside the field
And hear the dark
Slip of bodies,

The surge and swell
That remind us
We're never far
From all we love,

The dead never
Fully out of reach—

There is no relief from being God.

A dark and private weather

"And I experienced such great delight in gazing upon him (an angel) that I was compelled to forget the violent seizures that racked my whole body."
ST. ELISABETH OF SCHÖNAU (1129–1165)

This is how it happens.
The song that is not song
but the feathered sound of snow.
Like every piece of open sky
waiting for the one to worship,
the one to be worshipped.
Do not be deceived.
This is what it is to step
into the center of things.
And we were born for it,
this music, this shadow,
this shaggy downpour of words
that opens the door to the other
world where if you stare long enough
you can walk back into breath
and forget the dark sun setting.
The bones on fire. The thousand
lost days. And be gone

That winged and sacred thing

"And she sighs so deeply that her body is awakened and asks, "Lady! Where hast though been? Thou comest so lovingly back, so beautiful and strong, so free and full of spirit. But thy wanderings have taken from me all my zest, my peace, my colour, all my powers."
MECHTHILD OF MAGDEBURG (1207–1282)

Once there was a boy named Peter
who became a question:
How many worlds have been lost
in the peeling of an orange,
hands sticky with citrus,
juice sliding down your fingers?
How many selves split
by the sound of trees that daily
fall? In which version of this life
do you break inside of listening?

They were all the same question,
and they were the only way
he knew to empty himself,
to let the field move through him
and not the other way around.
It's not nearly as crazy as it sounds.
Imagine the huge stone of your body.
Picture what it is to live
with half the world swallowed
in that stone. Let the darkness grow
until you stand alone outside of it.
Watch as your life gets smaller.
Soon it will be nothing at all.

The crowd in the mind

*"I was in a very depressed frame of mind one Christmas night, when I
was taken up in the spirit. There I saw a very deep whirlpool, wide and
exceedingly dark; in this abyss all beings were included, crowded together,
and compressed."*
HADEWIJCH OF BRABANT (EARLY THIRTEENTH CENTURY)

I am the opposite of open space—
a field of a thousand buried,

a webbed and dusty corner filled with flies,
a back porch where wet leaves cling

as they rot in the patina of dusk
until 10,000 bits of slimy muck

cry the 10,000 names of the divine.
And half embedded in this loam,

we struggle into a sleep so deep
we dream of things larger than knowing,

where the present is merely a dark room
we assumed was locked tight, and all we need do

is listen to the night like a lover
begging for a chance to spring open.

That we might come back whole

*"When people said to me that I was demonically possessed so that I couldn't
stop myself, I was very ashamed, and I too said the same, that I was ill
and possessed."*
BLESSED ANGELA OF FOLIGNO (1248–1309)

I'm living someone else's life, where I'm
almost satisfied with all my choices.

It's not difficult to do, just pour yourself
through the space between long gaps of wanting,

the way you might pour milk into a jar.
The hands are yours. The arms are yours. The space

where you've been—
gone. To live in another's body is

paradise. Though it's not easy to stay put.
The flesh has its own curiosities—

to see your shadow cast by someone else,
to catch a glimpse of your old life coming

in and out of focus through the narrow lens
of waking dreams, to hear your name called

by the one you'd loved. There is no thread
to lead you back. Given that, it's easy

to lose your way, to lose everything
you've known about this sky until nothing

is left. No thing shines, and nobody knows,
including yourself, who or what you are.

Aglow, in silence

"He who does not believe in the words of Na Prous shall die an eternal death."
NA PROUS BONETA (1290–1325, BURNED AT THE STAKE)

You sit in your favorite chair, reading
a book, unable to trust the voice rising

from deep inside. You think that silence
will protect you from the poisonous dark

that permeates all you thought you knew.
You wish to move beyond your words into

another life, but what if that life is
as empty as your words, as empty as

a mouth agape, wanting to speak, wanting
to empty itself of the heat within?

You sit in your chair, not knowing where or
when your day will end, only that the world

grows thick with pain while you wait, your body
a slow fuse smoldering, when you could speak

words dripping with flame. Don't mumble your way
toward the sound of your own beginning.

To live means to cast the demon chained within
onto the ashes of your own silent pyre.

This creature

"Between the dread she had, of damnation on the one side and of her confessor's reproof on the other, this creature went out of her mind."
MARGERY KEMPE (1373–1439)

Between the glimpse of herself as a stranger
       in a passing mirror and the voice of the betrayed
              lover, this creature has forgotten her own light.

Between the night with its invisible shoals of longing
       and the circling of vultures in a summer sky,
              this creature fears to shake off her own name.

Between drifting in the calving light of dusk
       and the self-inflicted cuts of the soft ticked dark,
              this creature yearns for the story of another body.

Between the almond trees flowering outside her bedroom
       and the tongues of thirsty dogs waiting for certain knowledge
              of the world, this creature knows that everything

Is always spinning, that we are all circling around
       the gaping hole in the day, a vast ancestry of atoms
              stirring, a song of bodies filled with weeping.

As if the night had not begun

"In three days I shall become very ill and in thirty-four days I shall die."
MAGDALENA BEUTLER OF FREIBURG (1407–1458)

To have that kind
of certainty, to want

more than to begin
in rain, to believe

the sky is empty
and you the only light.

I don't even know when
or if I sleep,

or if I only think
about sleep.

Most of the time my body
turns wrong,

each night long enough
to endure,

each day something less
to lose.

There is a coffin
in which we wait—

the body still,
the heart still living,

the voice unwilling
to speak the truth

of that spider
webbing the dark corner—

our lives are mostly
distraction.

III

THE RENAISSANCE

"Men are so necessarily mad, that not to be mad would amount to another form of madness."

PASCAL

Flies in summer

"The air is not so full of flies in summer as it is at all times of invisible devils."
ROBERT BURTON

The definition of "possession" meaning possessed by a devil or demon is relatively recent, first appearing in 1580. Witch hunts were not medieval phenomena eclipsed by the rise of science and reason but rather a renaissance practice sponsored by science and so called "reason." The height of these hunts coincided with the establishment of the Royal Society of London in 1660. Because mental illness was seen as an occupation of the body by an outside force, treatment focused on ridding the body of these evil spirits through purging, sweating, vomiting, blood letting, and, in the most severe cases, destroying the body outright to save the soul. In one such case, a man who believed he was possessed by a wolf, had all his limbs chopped off to release him from the occupying spirit. He died as a result.

The deft spider spins

all those trembling selves beneath

a broken window

This imagined world

"It is well with me only when I have a chisel in my hand."
MICHELANGELO (1475–1564)

Only when this long dark throat opens
and the path through the forest speaks of rain

Only when the body is a garden waiting
to be turned, and nothing remains

but voice the day after it breaks
into leaves.

What else if not sky to remind us
of our need to drive and drive

until our lives are recalled to pain?

Only when the wound of want festers
to a certain silent clarity

can we stumble through this sliver
of emptiness and love the secret parts

of this imagined world.

In waning light

Where the sun bends
it shatters.

Where the body breaks
it speaks.

There is no measure
that keeps our silence,

no glad noise to mark
the dark, starved places

that blur our being.

Once I was eager
to remain

behind the door
that blocks the light,

content to peer through
the cracks into

the sound of others
pain.

Do not think, beloved
that I will do so, again.

We are made of more
than endings

and tangled years.

There are sicknesses that cure
the sick,

crimes that reconcile
the criminal to himself.

Only when the wound
opens can we bend.

In every heart, a mouth

"I thank it. More, I prithee, more. I can suck melancholy out of a song, as a weasel sucks eggs. More, I prithee, more."
JAQUES, *AS YOU LIKE IT*

Me next. Put me in line to welcome this tangle of worlds, this steady pull of empty days. Place the knife in my hand so that I may slice open the word-fruit, catch the juice in a bowl. Toss me before the need that swells the night, and I will eat, and if my mother calls out in worry, no matter. Nothing will keep me from un-seaming this turkey and seeking the obscene question within. In every heart there is a mouth, and this mouth is not afraid to open.

Absence

"Howl, howl, howl, howl."
KING LEAR

A coyote's howl announces, "I am here,"
or "stay away" depending on

our memory of the folding night
and the fickle call of weather—

enemy or friend. The deafness of trees
in winter reminds us that words fall away

the moment we find them. What silence wants
is to carry what we cannot across

the crack between earth and sky that threatens
to swallow each cry of our wounded lives.

We wonder how to get through most days,
searching for something we lack the language

to name, barely knowing how much of ourselves
we can take, afraid to ask how much will remain.

These distracted things

We must not believe in the words we bring
to silence,

    and the things we wish to write but lose,
    the moment we reach for a pen.

We must not believe in asking questions
of the sky

    and seeking answers in the scurry of black
    wings,

Like the mystery of why the night gets bigger
the darker it gets,

    or why the dog circles three times
    before lying down,

or why I covered my eyes
the first time you took off your clothes.

    We must believe in the strength of the dead
    insects that hold tight to our windshield

and in the broken strand of web
spinning in the air

    and in the way leaves in fall pretend
    to love the ground,

and that small hands will be enough.

This small knowing

"You do not know my heart. . . I am as clear as the child unborn."
REBECCA NURSE (1621–1692)

You do not know how one of my lives
can leak into another,

until nothing remains so
everything must be invented.

You do not know how the skin
slackens and the center goes soft

until not even the brittle bones
of birds can carry my song.

You do not know the desires
of even the oldest stars

or the secrets lying in the empty
hearts of the dead as they curl

like a leaf in morning's laundered light.

It is impossible to tell what lives
inside us when day turns to dusk.

I could say that I am haunted
by a field grown still after rain,

or that I am a mouth translated
into a tongue I cannot name,

or that I am as clear as an unborn
child, but that won't keep you from

wrapping this small knowing in rags again.

The sting of the finite

"I do not know [but] that the devil goes about in my likeness to do any hurt."
SARAH OSBORNE (1643–1692)

You do not have to be haunted
to forget your boots before

running through television snow,
or become a door blown open

by wind, or shove the ones you love
over the bannister and down

the spiral staircase at midnight.

You do not have to be dead
to summon friends by false names,

luring them to unsound bridges,
or call crows to weave pieces

of another life into nests
of regret that rest gently

on their unsteady heads.

The seasons where we are lost,
trapped deep in the forest

of ourselves while the moon sharpens
its edges, bear counting.

Don't rely on lessons learned from frost
that beards the trees in winter,

like a veil over the face of God.
This body is your own.

A different kind of dark

It's easy to find ourselves
in a different kind of dark
where we turn away from
the burn of knowing anything
for certain—who we will love
today, or how we will get up
in the morning, or when the long
whispering will end.

We stare at a candle, waiting
for whatever answer may come,
as if we could chart the blinding
roar of stars, when all we need do
is step through the mirrored door
that bends our eye back on the
nothing within. The far country
where few travelers have ever been.

Waking

"They called me mad, and I called them mad, and damn them, they outvoted me."
NATHANIEL LEE (1653–1692)

My first memory is of driving the school bus
my father restored. He fitted it with bunk beds,
a kitchen and bath, then painted it dirt brown.

We drove it cross-country, when I was four,
determined to leave the Minnesota cold
in search of anywhere without mosquitoes.

I still don't know where we were when I woke,
only that fog crawled off the lake and through
the haunted woods, and in that moment,

my life was not my life, and whoever said
we are not alone ever was lying because
the darkness shaped itself like a snake

coiled about the bus, swallowing every
color so that I didn't notice the lone light
shining from the cabin on the far shore.

I woke my younger brother and told him
our parents had been eaten by a rhinoceros.
He didn't bat an eye, as I explained

how I would drive the bus to the nearest town
and seek out a fireman with whom we could live.
The keys rested on the dash. The headlights burned.

My parents tell me they arrived before
I started to drive toward salvation—
they'd been spending the evening in that cabin

with friends—but I remember the narrow
road framed by rain stretching in front of me,
the terror of it, and the beauty.

IV

THE ENLIGHTENMENT

"Setting the sick apart sustains the fantasy that we are whole."
ROY PORTER

After the leaves fall, the black birds lift one by one

The history of madness is the history of power. The Great Confinement—as Foucault called it—begins in the late 17th century, reaching its height in the 18th, the rise of asylums coinciding with that of prisons, as the mentally ill were often housed with prisoners—a practice that continues today. Asylums served three functions, none of which had anything to do with treatment: Keep the mad confined to avoid familial shame; Contain the "terrible ulcer upon the body politic" (Diderot) so that the contagion of madness doesn't spread; And provide a site for spectacle where the populace could pay a small fee to watch the mentally ill sit chained to a cold floor, wallowing in their own waste.

Unstrung by silence

the harp of our body plays—

bare branch in the wind.

Too much world to hold

Remember, you are bigger than the hand
of God, which only holds so much dripping.

Your arms calve like glaciers dragging shadows
deep into the eclipse of some other moon.

You kick over each forgotten mountain
looking for the secret to jailing sky.

So why listen to the invisible
strangle of sounds rising from the trembling

grass? Why ask to live in yet another
starving dream where we trace our haunting

to absent notes of rain and the murky light
of dusk leaking through the kitchen window?

The only fixed point is black. The only
road back bannered in the animal's fur.

The dredging

And what we remember could fit on the flat
of a black moth's wing, could fall in the rustle
of leaves, flicked raw by the wind, of which
there is no end, from which, we invent what
we need, and what we believe lies fathoms
deep along the bottom of rime covered seas.
With starfish curtains sewn across our eyes,
we pour into the unmapped water,
that rising tide of blood-dimmed memories
and old-song bodies that surround us
like the dreams of thieves, of everyone
who ever tried to exist and failed,
and pull from there each bent and rusted nail
driven into the immense silence
we dare not touch, that unseen universe
that makes imagination's crown.

[I'm convinced I'm never awake]

"I have had a terrible night—such a one as I believe I may say God knows no man ever had. Dream'd that in a state of the most insupportable misery I look'd through the window of a strange room being all alone, and saw preparations making for my own execution."
WILLIAM COWPER (1731–1800)

I'm convinced I'm never awake. How else to explain this dream that sticks like wet leaves to the red tile floor inside the kitchen door? This dream where laughter curls beneath autumn's heavy rain, and the horizon at dusk lowers itself to let in more than one name, and I rise each day invented by a shiny new accident that looks and sounds in every way like something I have lived before and will again: I have a family, I have been in a family, I have a father, I have been a father, I have a son, I have been a son. And each and every one is complicit in choosing a mouth that fails to warn us that the man lying in bed who can't sleep and the boy lying in bed who can't wake are the same. The verdict guilty. Ready. Take aim.

The cut of feathers

Look how they go on without us,
the birds, or their shadows.

See how light entering the body
makes a kind of music, or nearly does.

Then close your eyes as if willing
yourself toward blindness,

as when saying goodbye to someone you love,
knowing you'll never see them again,

or leaving your child in a mental hospital
against her will.

The sound of everything unsaid
whispering through the trees,

like the pleasures we must invent,
in order to pretend to believe

we can make it through another day.
Where are you now as fists outgrow skin?

The body contains its bruises
like a world turned inside out,

or a stranger coming to the door,
one you'd swore you'd never see again.

Song of water and earth

This small drowning begins with the body,
how it carries what goes unspoken .

It begins with rain, and the memory,
not of the first drink that chokes

but of the last that fills the throat
like a lover's words retched from the past.

There is no limit to the ways we close
at night or the way morning breaks into

our calendared brains like a thief, or god,
dragging each childhood name back into light,

the day's pinch of air barely enough
to last us through hesitant dusk,

like the time they uncovered that boy,
the one trapped all afternoon inside

the gully's wall at the edge of the schoolyard,
a dark tunnel of his own making.

Lips blue, teeth clenched, fingernails lined
with unredeemable dirt, a miracle

he survived. The teacher asked,
back in class, if he'd wanted to die.

He burst into tears while I sat
still as stale air, wondering

how deep we must dig when
the world's more than we can bear.

All hunger and thumbs

"The idea of God is the sole wrong for which I cannot forgive mankind."
MARQUIS DE SADE (1740–1814)

You could stand quiet in the dark, waiting
for the Voice folded away in a drawer,
if only you knew what to do with your hands.

You could choose to give up whatever choice
you thought you had, sit down on the back
of a black sun and ride it into the scrub.

The problem is God's not an abstract noun
but found in every soggy smear of light
in which, by way of pain, we find ourselves
and drown.

Whose body is not torn

*"In the universe, there are things that are known, and things that are
unknown, and in between there are doors."*
WILLIAM BLAKE (1757–1827)

You have to stand in the darkness
Of a crucified moon

To know that what you see
Both is and is not there

You have to close your eyes
To hear the smoke rising

Like missing pages of music
From the next life and the last

You must learn to unravel
The shadows from your own hand

To feel the deeper wound,
That resurrection that reminds us

Nothing is ever ended,
That we are always, almost dead

You have to find your own way
Through the crack beneath the door

As for me, I believe
We are like little gods

Until morning takes us
And we retreat like dew

To sing and begin again

"I only live in my music."
BEETHOVEN (1770–1827)

You want to believe music will save you,
but there are too many lives to hold,

not counting the ones in which you do not
yet exist. And so you empty yourself

of blown open silence as the world
continues to burn, unattended.

Take the humming in the fields. Take the fugue
of trees and weeds that crown into this world

unredeemed, take the dirt that rescinds
our loneliness and the rain whose cadence

measures the hollow curve at the end
of our loves. It isn't enough to pluck

the ghosts of former selves we find wading
through the teeming grass. Not enough to walk

the unstrung roads sounding out who we are,
who we might have been, when all we need do

is listen to the drip of the world-song,
no matter the language, as it spills over

this lip of sky. The body and its rope
of notes like stars our eyes can't see.

This void

"Oh, this void, this terrifying void I feel in my breast!"
WERTHER (1774)

Ghosts surround us like trees
planting emptiness inside,

sorrows in parentheses
lapping at the body's last music.

Do you remember the ravaged love
of starlings,

how they still manage to thread
the final hourglass of sunlight

into a moon quilled with slivered glass?

Can you see the grass jeweled
with October's frost,

how the surface of things shines
with the silent mist

of this buried life,

the thousand desires
we keep from ourselves.

Into isn't

"I am—yet what I am none cares or knows."
JOHN CLARE (1793–1864)

There are places that have no name,
Where the wind stops midway through

The untranslatable night,
Static mixes with song,

And sometimes I know you.

Between one language and another,
No one remembers the silence,

And which rain erases which face, or why
The dark stream churns back toward childhood,

Where sometimes you know me.

All our instants thread through the not until
Every thing breaks into isn't

And we wake unhinged from all we knew,
Bodies screaming with stolen light,

The forgotten distances between us
Consumed by fire,

Until every thing is a shining.

All that we remember is wind

After Charles Wright

"The breath of heaven that sustained me was withdrawn, and I sunk into mere man."
THEODORE WIELAND (1798)

There's no clean getaway,

feathers in a frenzy,

into the sun.

from shoulders

of air,

despair nested

of the tallest tree,

with a papery tongue.

and blur,

to the broken,

sees his father's reflection

just before he flies

no Icarus,

making it this time

No wings budding

or lives woven

as if we could keep

in the branches

or stop words spoken

Like birds made of blood

we flock back

as when the son

in the window

into it.

V

THE NINETEENTH CENTURY

"If there is a universal mind, must it be sane?"
CHARLES FORT

Stealing fire

Madness as gift and punishment, as part and parcel of what it means to
be human. The fire stolen from the gods and the punishment for that
theft. Prometheus the symbol. William Blake the torchbearer. Blake who
courted madness. Blake who was never committed to an asylum
but whose career was built on the myth that all creativity is irrational,
all artists touched by flame.

The wooden spoon broke

when Father tried to spank me,

voice wrapped tight in blame.

With its mouth full

"I became insane with long intervals of horrible sanity."
EDGAR ALLAN POE (1809–1849)

Everything has become birds
And I have nothing to say

A church of birds
Inside my ear

And all I can do
Is listen

As if I'm the memory
Of a tree

On fire

In the middle of the forest

The last gasp of moonlight
Before dawn

Torches the eye

And when I wake

If I wake

I ask with a voice
Of oceans

With a thousand mouths like waves
That crash and fall and speak

Of the enduring loneliness

Of the human flower
Inside the fruit

How do we hang on
To our one life

When each day we spill
The seeds

And that chirping chorus
In our heads

Eats the path home

Tomb of words

"My heart pounds sickeningly and I turn pale . . . I often feel as if I were dead
. . . I seem to be losing my mind."
ROBERT SCHUMANN (1810–1856)

Little by little, I have learned nothing,
Except how to beat on the tomb of words,

To raise the lid and discover the trap—
How close we are to the final womb.

Like the time I took the dare and slow-walked
The length of the spillway beneath the dam,

Touched the great iron door and thought I felt
The weight of water on the other side.

Somewhere under the day, there's a garden
Where ladybugs' larvae lick clean the world

We spin, as if we could find the road back
Through corpse-dreamed earth to half-forgotten names.

If I could swallow the night in its silence,
Root beneath the moon's murderous understory,

Who's to say the fall would not be endless?
Look. I'm speaking to you now.

It is, after all, about darkness,
Its slow creep, how with eyes weighed down by crows

We stagger toward the immeasurable
Distance. How, in order to be lost,

We must travel far beyond the tattered
Melody of our forsaken bodies.

The flower's throat

This texture of darkness   These footprints like holes   This balancing
over the sunken world of childhood   This unforgivable sadness   This
body-house of silence   These stone memories   This vanishing

Light of words webbed about hands   Lucid vein of heat in every wound
Ripped wide   Burnished violence of morning   Pinned to the music of
want   Map of the inner mouth

So far on the other side   The flower's throat   Open   Calling

Now daybreak comes

"As far as my own sickness is concerned, am I not infinitely more indebted to it than to my health? It is to my sickness that I owe a higher health . . ."
FRIEDRICH NIETZSCHE (1844–1900)

For a home to be a home,
        You need to breathe
A little darkness.

Like a nail that longs to be struck,
        Or a wet sheet wanting the dry air,
The body abides,

Candled in moments of change,
        The poetry inside
Climbing out one window,

Returning through another,
        While the cardinal cocks its head
On the seed-stained ledge,

As if it couldn't comprehend
        Why the song of our thoughts
Doesn't bend to the mute sun

Around which we orbit,
        Why we can't defy
The laws of physics,

Let fly one ghost for another,
        And like a drunken doctor
Prepping for his last day,

Take apart all we've made
        of ourselves.

Backwards into being

"There will always be times when you take leave of your senses."
VINCENT VAN GOGH (1853–1890)

Standing outside my voice,
The stinging stone inside
Becomes silence.

Walking the dream-woods,
The slow slide of body
Backwards into being.

I cannot say which ghost
Carries our stories
Beyond the darkened mirror,

Or why every word we speak
To the scrambled night
Becomes a lie.

I only know that morning rises
Like steam from a dog's piss
On the cold snow, and

The mind is a door
That makes us strangers
To ourselves.

Crossing over

"I is the other."
ARTHUR RIMBAUD (1854–1891)

I is
Bleeding

To exist

Is madness wisdom

Breath want

This long passage into
Morning is

A hole in the top of my head

Is drenched in

This ache is
Somehow

Outside it all

Is everything

A person wants

Is this voice

This bleating silence

This place

Where the rain lives

Is

What

We become

Through the keyhole

I'm breathing your darkness
my friend,
carrying your silence,

for the time when
you claim each nail
as your own.

But how will I know you
when I see you?

Things change so
in this room
of wounded air

where we wait all day
for news
from a greater world

spending our time
trading one broken object
for another.

And the musky scent of dusk
floats through the keyhole
of our eye
like a confession

and every shadow resembles
a piece of this window
we tear in the world,

and the only thing a wall
understands
is how to break one god
into many.

Everything has a price

"My whole life has been spent walking by the side of a bottomless chasm, jumping from stone to stone."
EDVARD MUNCH (1863–1944)

Leaping   Toward lost   Toward   I refuse   This

Morning   Where wakened birds   Fall   Like a crush

Of stars   And the door   Seems   So   Far

What I would not   Give   To sleep   The night sky

Pooling   Around   This   Seamless present   That cocoons

My larval   Body   From which flowers   Grow

Like shedding   Skins   Within which   Lies

Dormant   In a deep   Green forest   The sound

Of one   Hidden   Scream.

This hungry map

Inside, no room for breath. Outside, the unforgiving paths of rain,

And a muddy field everywhere around me.

By what mouth do I leave this city when the day is a distance I cannot cross?

What voice will scale this fearful tower when each translation gets lost?

How to answer the question of the body's walls,

This maze of rooms made from crippled echoes,

This endless hall of regrets where solitude drips

Into tiny rivulets that bloom into a river flowing

Through the long darkness between our shadows.

Think how to unfold this hungry map,

How to imagine an other tangled world

Where we could conjure a battering ram to storm

This armada of doors like arms and open.

That old story

"Alone, I often fall down into nothingness. I must push my foot stealthily lest I should fall off the edge of the world into nothingness. I have to bang my head against some hard door to call myself back to the body."
VIRGINIA WOOLF (1882–1941)

Because leaves speak,
It is always October,

Words yellowing to flesh,
Mouths oranging to

Will someone please happen
Will someone please

Become

* * *

The part of the shepherd

Stepping out of this forgetting and into

The wilderness we need

* * *

To wander

　　Through the hole

Where we pretend

　　Every step

Is a word

       Like expiation,

Like snow

* * *

Holding the few remaining leaves

That cling to the branches

Because the wind

* * *

Also forgets   what it wants to say

About how little difference there is

Between coming   and going

VI
THE MODERN ERA

"The answer to illness is not necessarily cure."
LAUREN SLATER

When the night sky blooms

The early twentieth century as the Dark Ages of mental health treatment: insulin comas, lobotomies, forced sterilizations, and electro-shock therapy. The modern era of pill-based psychiatry begins with the introduction of Chlorpromazine in 1954. By 1970 more than nineteen million prescriptions of antipsychotics are written annually. Over the same period, the Soviet Union uses the same drugs to punish dissidents and make them docile. Medicine for one is torture for another.

We squat on the lip

of a ten-story building

as if we could fly.

Attention Woolworth Shoppers

"*The world breaks everyone, and afterward, some are strong at the broken places. But those that will not break it kills.*"
ERNEST HEMINGWAY (1899–1961)

And we sat in rapturous exhaustion
on the spinning stools in the diner
at Woolworth's—every store had one—
attending to the mystery of donuts.
And we saw with fingers that gripped cracked
and chipped cups of coffee that the shortest
distance between the door you come in
and the door you go out was sitting right
here between the water-stained silverware
and the napkins on which we wrote prayers
before passing them to the tired and silent
waitress for absolution. And the wailing
of the PA across the vast dust
of unmopped aisles confirmed there was nothing
left to save. And the end caps hawked their wares
with the curled tongues of long-dead hucksters.
And still we listened, as if there were time
for their thin and hollow cry to reveal
the most treasured secrets of our anemic lives.

All that remains

"By daily dying, I have come to be."
THEODORE ROETHKE (1908–1963)

I work hard   to forget   myself   so I can sleep   We live so many
deaths   it's difficult   to see   the snow   blind   as we are   by mouths
moving   At some point   we stand inside   our own   absence   Emptiness
drawn taut   over the horizon   like a slow alphabet   of broken   glass
spread across   the floor   until   each shining shard   exhausts us,
until   all the moons   of our mistaken lives   dissolve   into fierce
And now   here   the depthless lake   all that remains.

There are all sorts of violence

*"Mine has been a life of such shame. I can't even guess myself what it must
be to live the life of a human being."*
OSAMU DAZAI (1909–1948)

You do what you can to touch everything
because it's hard to believe so much sadness

haunts the world, hard to see through the darkening
window that refuses to look back.

Do you remember how you arrived here?
The deep rain that washed away the stranger's

heart you will never know, the wind that cleaved
the long breath of your broken nights in two,

the light sinking like an itch forever
below the surface of your dying skin.

It's enough to stay the body's drowning,
yet you refuse to see our days are made

of frenzied waves hitting the shore,
spread so thin we forget what it's like

to imagine we exist. As if by
closing our eyes and looking through the glass

of half-remembered childhood we could spy
anything like the spirit close up.

[And so I wake]

"I find the greatest serenity in hallucination."
CLARICE LISPECTOR (1920–1977)

The dark threshold beckons. The drunken night demands I wash out
my eyes. The hour complicit in erasing the wall between what I know
and what I refuse to know. The only thing left is to search for an exit, to
travel into a language I don't understand. And so I wake to find my being
depends on standing. I rise out of the dream's slow dissolve, losing my
feet a little with each step, traveling further into all my gods dying like
cockroaches in the forgotten corners, wondering who, then, is the pilot
of this infested body.

Room of windows

*"God knows there certainly ought to be a window around here somewhere,
for all of us."*
RICHARD YATES (1926–1992)

You remember the room you had as a child
that overlooked the swing from which you jumped

into a pile of autumn leaves that fell
like little windows. You remember, too,

the tornado that formed above your house
then skipped down the street looking for doorways

into trees that would welcome the wind, or
sewer pipes that spilled into fields calling

you to crawl into womb-dark warrens
where you slipped between the error of days.

Whether the tenuous night stretches for miles
or opens to a room made of windows

and doors that take you always everywhere
depends on where you stand. It's there despite

the many drops of rain that sing against
the pane, saying yes, you, too, will be lost,

as if you were the window, the door,
the living wound that refuses to open.

The wind is an ocean

"Once I was beautiful. Now I am myself."
ANNE SEXTON (1928–1974)

Once, I was an eye
That looked toward
Morning's cry,

An ear breaking
Across evening's
Orange dissolve.

Now, I'm a mouth
Curled with earthworms,
Like murmurings
Over a castle wall.

I'm tempted to close
My body to this dream,
A deposed king
Seeking retribution.

Then, my son tornados
Through the house
Sucking up cookies,
The cat, a throw rug,

And I remember,
I, too, was once a boy
Feeding the other pool,

That empty self,
Whose only rule
Is to open, asking
To be filled.

All we wished to see

"I am terrified by this dark thing that sleeps in me."
SYLVIA PLATH (1932–1963)

I don't want to scare you,
but sometimes at night
my body opens.
I reach deep inside
and pull this thing out,
examine its moon-
flesh in the weak-coffee
dark, in the same way,
in more reckless times,
I pulled myself into
other days. It speaks
with a voice half mine,
half made of ashes,
like the shadows
of flying birds
that refuse to eat,
saying, you are not
here. You are not here.
This is water,
I say in return,
these are bones and
this night a small tin
painted with stars.
It cries and eventually
goes silent so I can lie
in peace and imagine,
as I hold it tenderly
in my hands, that this
is the world I'd
always wanted.

Dearest love

If I were still myself on this cold journey
through winter fields beneath a washed-out moon,

I might speak the night and its shiver of stars
or, even, the bent sky with its black fire.

If I were still willing to give up
every kind of pain that buries us,

I might speak of the thick river of bees
that runs within like a line of leaves

through autumn's waning light.

But I'm little more than a wraith drifting
through the darkness of this recurring dream.

How deep the need to tread the faithful
language of our bodies, to attend

the choir of emptiness demanding
we sing its covenant of knowledge.

It's how we give ourselves to this weaving,
we who have time to change so little, we

who have only begun to understand.

The gathering

*"Do I perform sometimes in a manic style? Yes. Am I manic all the time? No.
Do I get sad? Oh yeah. Does it hit me hard? Oh yeah."*
ROBIN WILLIAMS (1951–2014)

After the gathering
      of ghosts

swells the itinerant
      dusk,

and the turkey vultures
      sitting in trees

have claimed another day,
      and the cries of crows

cling to your clothes
      as the last light

leans in low,
      conjuring

the darkness that kisses
      your eyes,

the wound awakens,
      and you are left

to inherit the trembling
      slowness of the earth,

to once again feel
      your length

of breath about you
      circling, circling,

like a shadow
      over the winter grass.

For whom you are suffering

"I am mentally ill. I can say that. I am not ashamed of that. I survived that, I'm still surviving it, but bring it on. Better me than you."
CARRIE FISHER (1956–2016)

As if we could own
this madness, dissolve
it into liquid,
a tincture to take
twice a day, or pop
in pill form, as if
we needed something
to remind us one
fever dream is not
enough, the muddy field
empty as a scream
without sound, a silence
without ticking, a
body without—to
miss it is to grow
afraid, to pretend
to know the terrible
charity of words.
Better to leave,
than watch and wait
in the upstairs room,
eyeing the mirror
above the dresser
where we once
were caged,
like every delirious
bird twittering
on the edge

of their dark laughter.
No mouth, no matter
how small, should
be kept from singing.

Acknowledgments

After the Pause: "Room of windows"

Barrow Street: "Too much world to hold"

The Café Review: "Absence" and "In waning light"

Chiron Review: "Black Angel"

Contemporary Haibun Online: "After the leaves fall, the black birds lift one by one" and "Stealing fire"

Forklift, Ohio: "Waking"

The Gettysburg Review: "A dark and private weather," "That winged and sacred thing," and "Tomb of words"

Grist: "All we wished to see" and "Dearest love"

Haibun Today: "Flies in summer"

The Hollins Critic: "A different kind of dark"

Hotel Amerika: "In every heart, a mouth"

The Inflectionist Review: "All that remains," "Into isn't," and "There are all sorts of violence"

Lake Effect: "There is no shepherd but silence" and "This imagined world"

Main Street Rag: "All that we remember is wind," "Somewhere hidden," "The dredging," "The road out is like the road in," and "This void"

Negative Capability Press: "All hunger and thumbs," "Backwards into being," "Crossing over," and "This is how you become absent"

[PANK]: "Attention Woolworth Shoppers"

Permafrost: "The flower's throat"

Prairie Schooner: "With its mouth full"

Prism Review: "[And so I wake]," "Everything has a price," "The gathering," and "For whom you are suffering" (in slightly different form)

Redactions: Poetry and Poetics: "The cut of feathers"

RHINO: "The wind is an ocean"

Roanoke Review: "What certain voice"

Rock & Sling: "The crowd in the mind"

Stirring: A Literary Collection: "The biggest problems come from being" and "The sting of the finite"

The Summerset Review: "Aglow, in silence" and "As if the night had not begun"

Sweet—A Literary Confection: "To sing and begin again" and "This hungry map"

Unbroken: "A candle lit in the hollow of a wall"

Verdad: "[I'm convinced I'm never awake]" and "Through the keyhole"

The Worcester Review: "Now daybreak comes"

Special thanks to Betsy Johnson for her care in reading these poems.

PETER GRANDBOIS is the award-winning author of eleven previous books. His poems, essays, and short stories have appeared in over one hundred magazines and been shortlisted for the Pushcart Prize, Best American Essays, and Best American Horror. His plays have won the Best of the Neil LaBute Festival and have been performed in St. Louis, Columbus, Los Angeles, and New York. He is poetry editor at *Boulevard* and teaches at Denison University in Ohio. You can find him at www.petergrandbois.com.

CPSIA information can be obtained
at www.ICGtesting.com
Printed in the USA
LVHW030323210521
688044LV00004B/292

9 781944 467265